I0115833

BACK PAIN

Relief in 45 minutes

Marcus D. Norman

RoyceCardiff
Publishing House

Seventh -Edition

ISBN-13:978-0615973647

ISBN-10:0615973647

Digital Format ASIN: B008PYPC74

Printed in the United States of America

MarcusDNorman@gmail.com

Forward:

It has been my experience the simplest things in life can work out the best. In this area of back pain relief, you have a different option that you can add to the doctors, drugs and surgery routine. I will show you how you can do it. I'm going to tell you how you can take control of your back pain issues once and for all. I have more than 30 years involved in physical training with focuses on skeletal and muscular alignment. I had my own debilitating back pain issue and a mother who has a lifelong bout with back pain management and has gone through the normal medical model of doctors, pain meds, therapy and surgeries. Those observations had led me to put my ideas what really works in this one book. And now also a 10 part video series, which I have included free for your further benefit. Enclosed is some simple stretches and habit changes that you can do.

Imagine you up and running like never before!

This little book has made a huge difference for so many people, so at the end of this book I will ask you for a review that way others can find it and benefit from it.

Before you review it though, you have to read it :-)

So – let's get started.

Introduction:

If you have back pain, you could go see your doctor, or even a specialist. However, if there were a way to resolve the issue yourself, I believe it is great to do some simple exercises to relieve your pain and get long lasting results. Marcus Norman's simple guide "Back Pain relief in 45 minutes" is such a resource that provides you with those techniques and strategies to get you started.

My training is in dealing with human behavior and habits. One habit people with back pain have, is not taking their problem seriously. I recommend you start taking your back pain seriously and start to do the simple exercises as recommended in this book.

I wish you well with your back, and hope you soon will be feeling a lot better. That will also make you feel happier!

- Marc Veghters, B.Ed., U. Dip, Med., M.Sc.

Guarantee:

Practice the ideas in this book for 7 days and if you are not **thrilled** with the results. Simple request a full refund, No questions asked!

Table of Contents

My life was over!

My eyes opened, and I was looking at the ceiling. I had intense pain in my torso; I realized I could not move my body. When I attempted to move left or right, shooting pain ran through me. it was hard to breathe.

"Wow! it was amazing. I was frozen, trapped. What is happened?" I always thought I was very healthy and fit. I did regular exercises, hiking, yoga, biking, swam and had plenty of physical work. What happened? Oh no, my world is coming to an end. I have a business to run, what am I to do?

I picked up the phone and called a very dear friend Sandy. Sandy is my friend who studied physical alignment of the skeletal and muscular systems and a certified EMT. She is a bit of a study addict. Always taking classes to improve her knowledge and skill set to care for others. That is to our benefit.

She came right over and helped me get out of bed and onto the floor. Ouch!!! thought I was going to die!!!. She showed me a few movements. By that afternoon, I was back up walking again. However, my body was greatly twisted and distorted.

I had made a few phone calls, and it seems that the doctors recommended that I rest for 2 weeks and take pain medications. (Later I found out how 2 weeks can really set you back, you need to move your body that is what it is designed for). However that was not an option for me, I had a business and a life to get back to.

My mother had a back injury at work years ago; she went to the many doctors and had a few different surgeries, all promising improvement in her condition. Her condition got worse. They started my mom on heavy pain medications; until this day she still has to take pain meds, which affects her ability to function, and to think clearly to live a normal life. Her back will never be the same. One doctor admitted she would have been better off without any of the invasive surgeries. He also said that she most likely would have healed herself if they had given it more time and no surgeries. Mom's favorite thing is to go swimming, which she cannot do to the full extent. Needless to say, I was looking for other options than the standard modality of Doctors, Pain meds, Surgeries.

With the exercises from my friend and a few

things that I added from my experience in yoga, sport training and physical training, I was back to work in one week and fully recovered in a few shorts weeks!

HOW TO: BACK PAIN TREATMENT?

I have found and read many great books on how to heal your back. However, they are very long-winded with many explanations and a lot of information and histories that didn't really help to immediately repairing my back. My intention for this little tiny book is to give you enough information on what helped me and other friends and how to get you started on your journey to healing your back NOW! I will be giving you ideas on how to short-term and long-term repair of your back without all the fluff and filler. I will try to get to the point, so as you can get back to your life.

This is what this book is about, so let's get up and playing again, without any surgeries, doctors or drugs. Let's get started!!!

I can get you pain relief in the next 45 minutes; only jump ahead and go straight to relax stretch pose in the Lazy Man's Chair Pose chapter!!!

Also, you get immediate access to the "how to demonstration videos series" near the end of the book!

Some causes of back pain A Movement problem

I find it very important to understand that some of the things below you may be doing. However when you start feeling better but continue to keep doing the same things that caused the problem in the first place, you will get the problem again. So please take note of the suggestions below.

You cannot expect to do the same behavior and get different results!

Number 1: Chairs

Chairs are a 1st world disease in my opinion.

We sit at work, at home, in our cars, in front of the TV for many hours way too long, and we do not really move our bodies anymore. In our modern society, it is very easy for us to live in a box, and our motions are very limited. I've traveled and lived in many Third World countries and notice the people can be 90 years old, and they can still sit on the floor. I know some people over 70 who are still climbing trees to pick fruit. Do you know anybody in the First World, our modern society, that can climb a tree at the age of 70 and pick a 12 pound fruit?

One thing that I found very helpful and it’s this. I have a little cooking timer I set it for between 30 and 50 minutes when I'm working; at the end of my 30 to50 minutes, I set it for

10 minutes and I move around for 10 minutes. What do I do for 10 minutes? Well this is a bonus; I do my honey do list; I fix and take care of little details around the house. It can be anything like laundry, cleaning something, doing a small repair job I've been wanting to get to. My wife thinks I'm a Hero! When the timer goes off I get back to work another 30 to 50 minutes. Funny thing is that I get more done than sitting there for hours on end with no breaks.

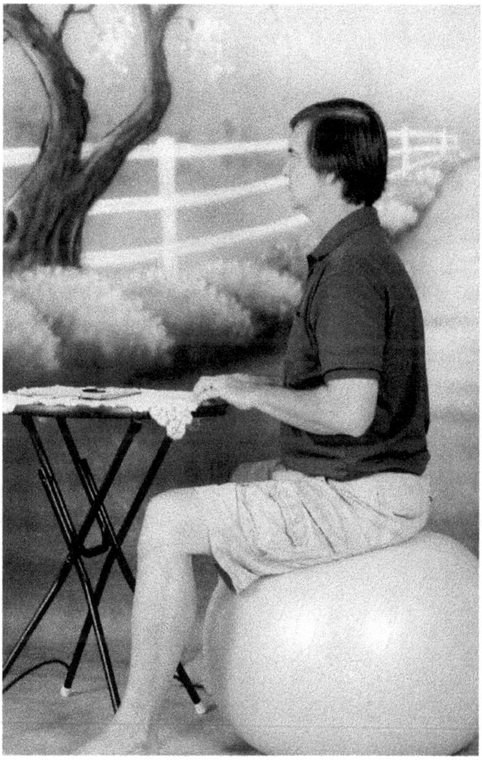

As Mickey said:

"Try it, you'll like it!"

When using a chair, sometimes part of my

body would go numb. Instead of a chair, I mostly use an exercise ball. It engages a lot more of my muscles in my body, also helps to keep the butt from getting flat. My legs stay toned. It also helps to build core strength and to keep the spine aligned! It helps me to look great, and it's Fun!

Number 2: Exercise

Regular cardiovascular and strength exercises are fine and should be done on a regular basis. However, I find that it is important in life is to do stretches. So implement some type of yoga or Pilates.

Number 3: Slumping forward

Does your head leaned forward? How about your shoulders, do they get rounded rolling forward? Some of the exercises I have enclosed start to correct this. However, there is much more you can do, which is not in scope of this book. See Pete Egoscue book "PAIN FREE"

Number 4: Poor Diet

It goes without saying a poor diet can lead to poor health and poor healing. This book is intended to be short and quick and give immediate relief for your back issues, so I don't need to go into any healthy diet ideas as that's easy enough to find out. Please note you must drink adequate amount of water also and stay away from high-fat high calorie diets. And if you're overweight you're putting extra strain on your skeletal and muscular systems.

Number 5: Shoes

Best not to wear shoes. As least as possible, go barefoot when you can. Don't wear shoes especially around your home or even at your office. If you can, take them off. Our bodies are designed not to wear shoes. Think about it - there are millions of years of evolution to perfect the amazing foot. Strapping our feet into 1 inch of foam rubber - do you think that's the way we are intended to walk? However, in our modern world we do need to wear shoes. So, if your shoes are worn out and leaning, replace. I don't believe in orthotics; they just exacerbate the issue with body posture and alignment. When you must wear shoes, use something like a FiveFingers shoe. It's very thin, like a sandal fits, like a glove over each toe. I find them amazing and FUN!!!

Number 6: Bed

I did not realize how important a good bed was till after I purchased one. I find high quality beds to be of great benefit. In my research, the beds with the air number system are very expensive glorified camping mattress, my butt pushed down the center, and my head and my feet were up in the air? What the heck!!!!!!! They let me try it for 90 days. When I returned it to the salesperson, I asked him how many people return these air mattress beds. He said more than 30%.

My personal bed now is a 100% latex bed. My latex is organic, healthy, and it lasts a long time and is not hot or cold. It's well worth the money.

Number 7: Smoking

People who smoke are 2 times more likely to have back pain than people who do not smoke. Smoking allows less oxygen into your body, so that poor health and slowing healing. Enough said!

Number 8: Bras

Women with large breasts – it's very important to have the correct supportive, comfortable bras. That way you will not pull on your back and your shoulder blades.

Number 9: Purses, bags, briefcases.

Carrying around a heavy item with one arm, or with one shoulder can lead to an imbalance in your posture. Also on another note, men should not put wallets in their pants pocket.

Number 10: Flip-flops

Do you love flip-flop shoes? I do. They are very convenient. However, you must curl your toes to keep them on your feet which pulls on a whole array of muscles which are not beneficial to your back. My recommendation is to ditch the flip-flops and buy some other kind of fun sandals without the thingy that goes between your toes.

Number 11: Stress and depression

For the stress, see chapter 3, solution number 1, relax.

For depression that is a significant subject. I've had experience with that. Doctors and Drugs did not help as they just made me a zombie. Da da da.... What I realized is that most everybody has up and downs in the month, that is pretty typical. What worked for me was getting my life in balance, correcting my diet, consistently eating and sleeping at the same time every day, as much as possible. Being aware of my moods. Most of all what I did was when I feel any little depression coming on, I would do some physical exercise or sport.

"The Doctor told me I would be on medication for the rest of my life."

Hog Wash to that! I have had no anti-depression medicines for more than 28 years! I have the most amazing lifestyle, if I was on any type of mood altering medications, that would not be the case.

Here's a book I recommend. you can get it at Amazon HAPPINESS PROJECT, proven shortcuts: by Jimmy Johnson

" **HAPPINESS PROJECT Hacked**

Proven ***shortcuts***:

Happiness Advantages,

Traps and Easy how to Allow **Radical** Self Improvement

to Happen to You, starting in the next 24 hours!

(Motivational, Self-Help, Personal Growth & Inspirational)

"Don't worry, be happy!"

-Bobby McFerrin

Yeah, I know what you're thinking: "Oh my gosh, many things I could do better". Don't feel guilty, that's not why I've brought these things up. We are just fine the way we are. It has come to my understanding we (me) are not broken and need no fixing. That said here are some suggestions that you may want to do to improve the quality of your life, or you could look at it this way, now you have another reason to do them. For every action, there is a reaction. So what action would you like to see different in your Life?

Remember, life is good and gets better every day!.

Okay, let's get into the meat of the subject.

Back Pain Management

1. Relax:

My chiropractor said I was a wreck; I needed to relax, too much work and stress and not enough downtime no balance in my life. He told me when you have a full lifestyle and too much going on, it will come out in one of two areas. You can go mentally crazy, or your body will start to complain and show signs.

Before doing these back pain exercises, you may need 1 to 2 days of bed rest, 48 hours max, doing nothing , turn off the work phone, catch up on watching your favorite movies and popcorn.

My favorite popcorn recipe:
Fine ground cayenne pepper and nutritional brewer's yeast flakes.

Really it's very good, check it out.

Okay, how about reading your favorite books, that's fine. I love my Kindle reader!

Soak: Take as many hot baths as it feels good with Epson salt and baking soda; a little aromatherapy with lavender oil is also a benefit for relaxing.

2. Ibuprofen:

Dr. Victor said I could take the maximum dosage of ibuprofen for many days without any adverse effects. Ibuprofen can reduce swelling, which reduces pressure, hence reducing pain. Okay, I know I said no drugs; however I think ibuprofen is very mild with little to no long term effects. If you don't want to, you don't have to. My back pain was so high that it was difficult to breathe fully. I took it for the first two days.

3. Breathing:

Breathe from your belly and not your chest. This will get you centered in your body, improving your oxygen intake. This type of breathing is taught in martial arts, yoga and centering activities. Also, an additional breath that will help you heal, see chapter 4 for the Darth Vader exercise breathing.

OK, now you are on your way! Should be feeling somewhat better. The next few chapter is a simple back pain exercise routine I developed to get me back to 100%!

let's go amigo!!!

Darth Vader Breathing

This is really an energizing thing to do once you get the hang of it. Inhale slowly through your nose and exhale through your mouth. When exhaling, produce the sound HHHHHHAAAAAA. Next, keep your mouth closed while exhaling. Create the same sound as before, though, this time with your mouth closed. The position of your throat is unchanged and natural. Make sure the sound originates from the throat and not from your nose.

Now maintain the same throat sound position

while inhaling, producing the same murmuring sound. (Darth Vader)

Feel your heartbeat. Inhale over approximately 3 to 5 heartbeats and exhale over the same amount.

This may take a little practice. Notice the development of your oxygenated blood flow. You will feel energized. More free and light. Great to do when you are tired also.

Enjoy!

Kitchen Counter Stretch

This is very easy to do, gives you a deep stretch, and it feels soooooooo good. I was taught this by a 70-year-old snow skier at a beautiful mountain Lodge in Upstate New York. I was skiing with New York's finest, The New York City Police on their annual ski trip, Great Fun! It sure made a significant improvement in my flexibility for the days of learning how to snow ski.

Stand facing the kitchen counter. Place your palms on the counter shoulder width apart walked back into your heels. Torso and legs should be at 90 degrees. Feel the stretch through your arms and your hips are in line with your heels and your feet parallel and hip distance apart. Do this pose for 3 minutes including the Darth Vader breathing. Let your head and buttocks relax and your belly arch toward the floor.

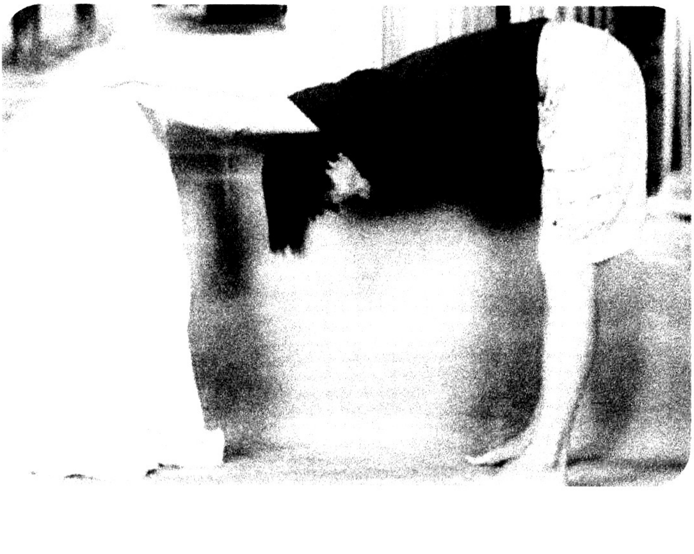

Lay-down Twist

Yes, this one is easy to do, other than feeling good! Enjoy it . Feel free to stay in the pose longer if you like. Sometimes I do it when I watch a movie. Many years ago, one of the Top Hang Glider pilots in the World, my friend Chris Perkins he showed me this pose. At the time, I was cleaning carpets and flying gliders; it was greatly appreciated relieving tension in my back.

Lie down on the floor on your side with both knees together to form a right angle to your body. Extend your arms out level with the shoulders and, parallel with the bent knees, and put your palms together. Take your top arm and put it over on the other side, face your head with your eyes looking toward the ceiling to start. When it starts to become more comfortable, turn your head in the opposite direction of your knees. That way you receive a deep stretch. Do the Darth Vader breathing, relax and notice the feeling as if you are melting into the floor. If there were a goal, it would be to let both shoulders lie flat on the floor. Do this for at least 5 minutes per side, as you start to loosen up you may most likely need to readjust shoulders and knees.

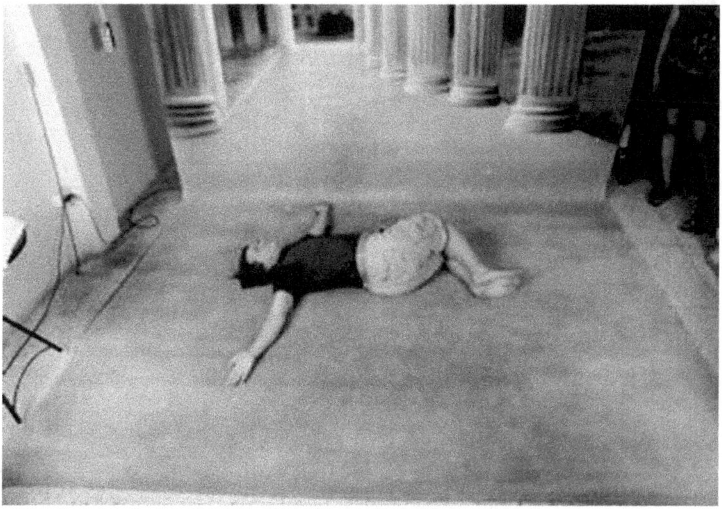

Lazy Man's Chair Pose

My 4 foot 11 inch tall, 88 pound wife used to do certified nurse assistant work. One afternoon when I picked her up, she was in so much pain at Wally's world, my wife had to use the electric wheelchair to go shopping. It took all her power just to walk to the front door of the Wal-Mart Store. With just 2 days of this chair exercise, she was happily back at work. She loves me even more now:).

Lie on your back with your legs resting on the seat of a chair or a large collection of cushions. Use some pillows under your legs if needed to adjust the height. Put your arms out at 45° with your palms up. Do the Darth Vader Breathing deeply and slowly from your belly; be aware of your back relaxing. Let yourself melt into the floor until both left and right sides are flat on the floor; this may take up to one hour. If you do over one hour at a time, it has no additional value, and in fact it could be detrimental. If you have a lot of pain the first few days, you can do this a few times per day. Leave a few hours in between. Once you are well, you can do maintenance or weekly tune up. I do 15 minutes; You can do as little as 5 minutes and feel the benefits. Sometimes I take a power nap in this position; it's get me more focused, free up my body, and I feel great!

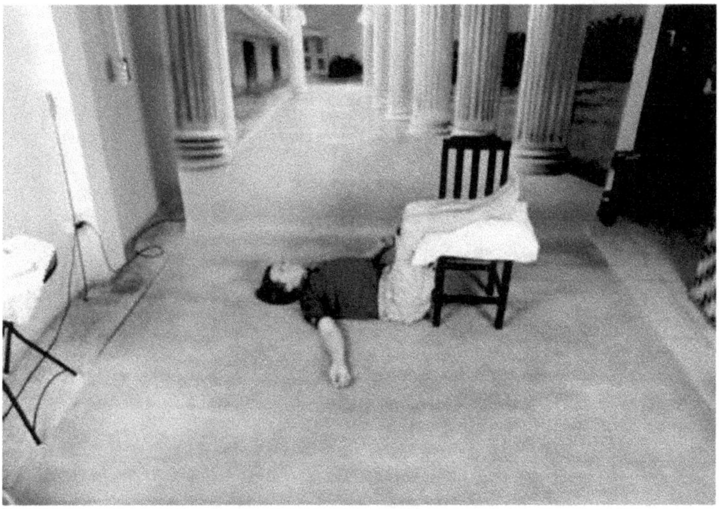

The life saver

Level Groin Stretch

This is a position that my friend Sandy showed me that really saved my life. It brought my twisted body back into balance.

Just because this position is easy to do, don't be fooled by the great benefits you will receive, you have some large muscle groups that are very tight, so be patient,

Lie on your back with one leg bent at a 90° angle resting on a chair, and the other leg set on the top of the 4th level which is the same level as your bent leg. These levels can be made from a small step ladder stack of books or something similar. The idea is to remain in this position until your back is relaxed and flat on the floor; this may take up to 40 to 50 minutes per position. Repeat on the other side at the same height. **Important** to do both legs at the same level before you move down. Then move your way down the levels until you end up on the floor. Two important things here.

Number 1: Keep the elevated foot relaxed and pointing up, don't allow it to flop over, use books, sandbag or blocks.

Number 2: Your back must be flat on the floor before moving to the next level.

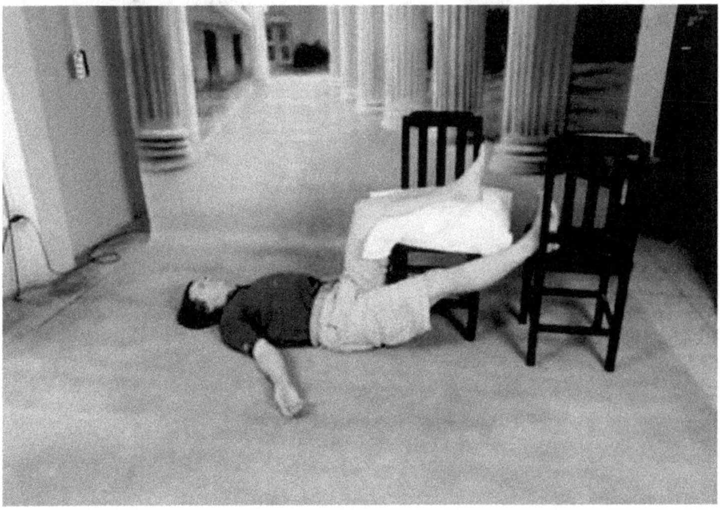

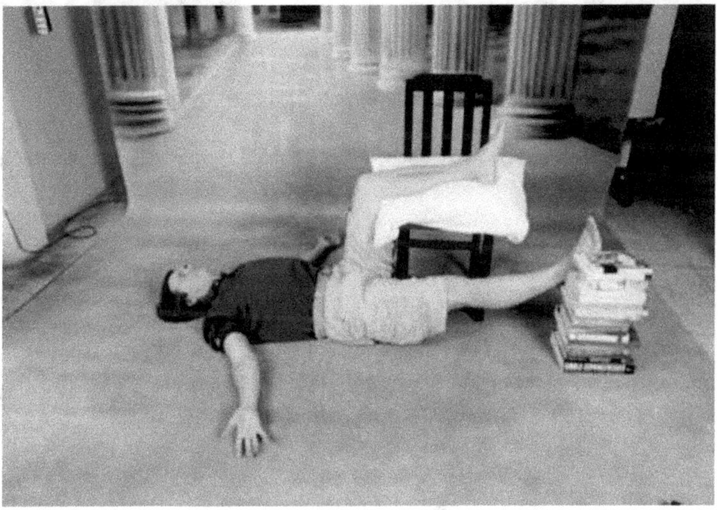

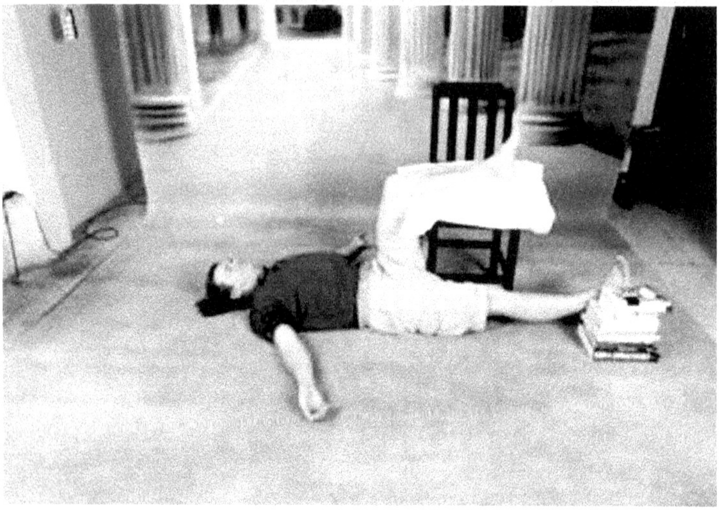

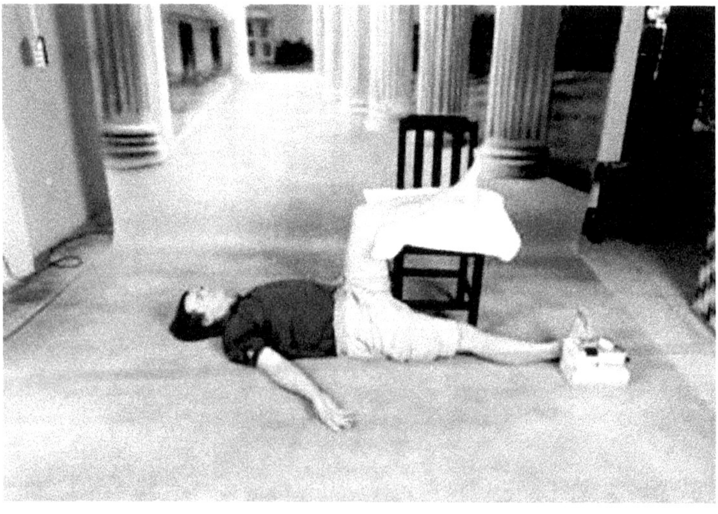

Oh Shit!

How you eliminate affects your health forever!

Okay, here is the OH SHIT part. Do you realize that the way that you eliminate has been affecting your health for your whole life? Our fancy Western toilets nicknamed thrones are unnatural as they don't let the body fully stretch out and don't allow us to eliminate completely which can cause a multitude of challenges for our physical bodies. More information is available on the benefits of proper elimination. But to keep this brief you can get further knowledge at the BackPainReliefin45minutes.com where you can watch a short clip about it. One important point is you can get a stretch in your daily bowel movement. Really!

When I was in Santa Fe New Mexico visiting a chiropractor for a checkup, I was using the facilities to go to the bathroom. There was a picture on the bathroom door: it showed a person squatting on the toilet! It explained the benefits and why. This was also confirmed by a doctor, most of the world evacuates, has a bowel movement, goes number 2, or whatever you'd like to call it. in a squatting position. People in Third World countries squat to do their duties. They have a lot fewer challenges with back issues than first worlders who use the throne type toilet.

I even convinced one of my yoga teachers Dave (who by the why was a semi-pro volleyball player)who was having issues with his back. Dave's lower back was frozen, locked up with very little movement. It affected his yoga practice, volleyball and sex life also. He really wanted it back pain cure. I encouraged him to give it a go. He saw vast improvements with his back by only going to the toilet like most of the world. Even though he did yoga 6 days a week, this simple idea changed him forever!!! Oh, he's wife thanked me very much also, if you know what I mean!

Note: Most of the world uses a squatting position for social time, conversation and, or business. Many countries that I have visited in Asia and South America have no chairs. It is very common to go to the market and squat when purchasing your fruits and vegetables. At first, I found this very difficult for my Western body. My ankles and calves were not used to this stretch. No way were my heels going to touch the ground!!!! Yikes!!! However I found it amazing once I got used to it. I found it natural, and it's a relaxing way to socialize. So if you are like me and have this wonderful Western body that is not quite as flexible as our friends in the Third World, please make sure that you do the preparation and warm-up exercises before you move on to squatting on Western toilet. It may take a few weeks for your muscles to loosen up.

If not you will find it very difficult and maybe even dangerous; imagine slipping off the toilet.

Really! Enjoy!

Preparation and warm-up Exercises:

Stand with your feet parallel slightly wider than your hips in your bare feet. Bend your knees and lower your hips down toward the ground. Relax your shoulders. If your heels don't touch the ground, like most Western men. Simply put some books or towels on your heels to support you. The idea is to work your way up to 5 Darth Vader breaths, with your heels flat on the floor. Place your palms together it in front of your heart. Work on lifting your head toward the sky, straightening your back. Next, move an elbow to the opposite knee as in the photo below. You can put a little pressure on the twist. Sometimes my back makes a cracking sound, that is good! it is just getting your parts straight! Then do the other side with the twist also.

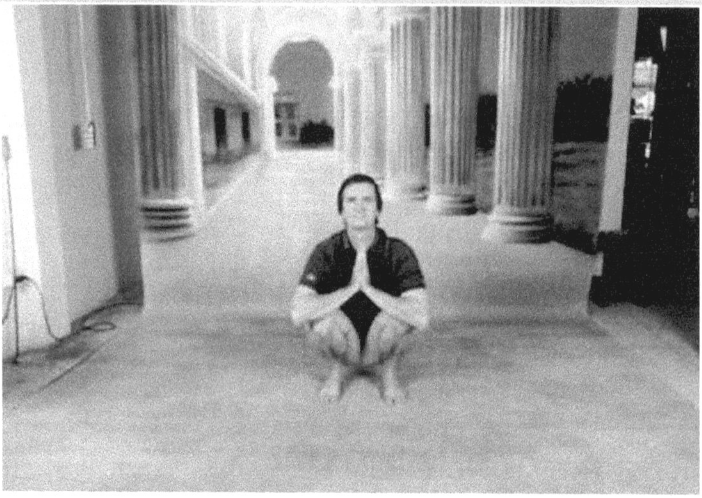

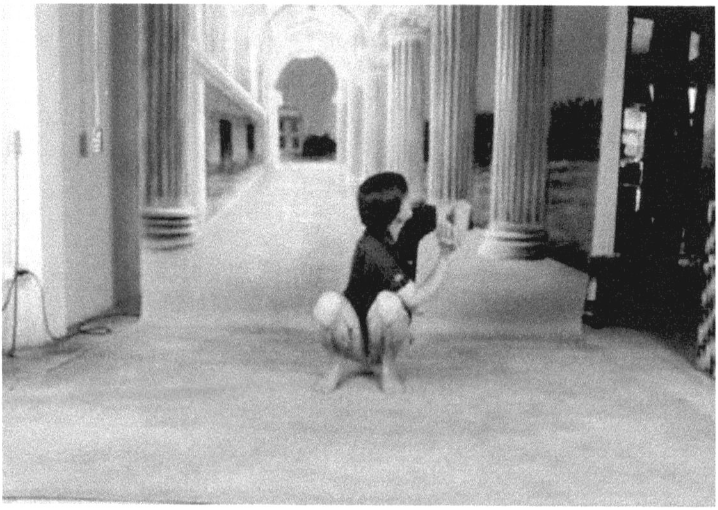

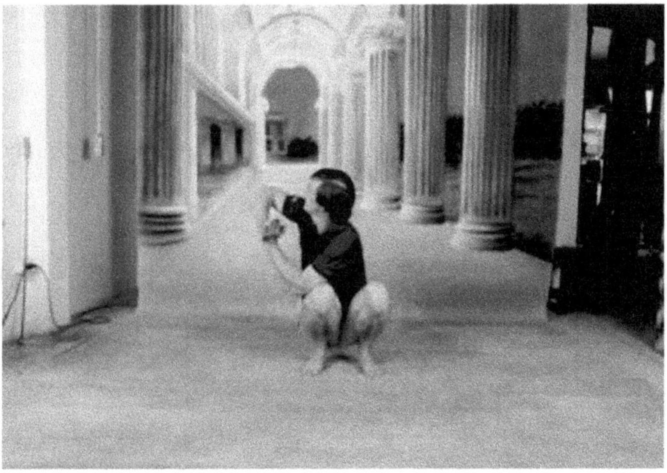

Benefits:

Stretching out the tight western calf muscles, also helps to stimulate your digestive system which helps to relieve constipation. Helps pregnant women open their hips. Relaxes the nervous system, improves concentration, stimulates circulation, helps your breathing, develops your lung power and is a nice deep relaxing backstretch.

Basic method for squatting on a Western toilet:

if you're of average size and weight , it's best to lift up the toilet seat. Put 1 or 2 hands on a wall or something to hold you steady as you put one foot on the rim of the bowl, (no I don't touch the wall or use any support anymore, have been doing this for years, see advance method below) gently and slowly repeat with the other foot. Be Very Careful Not to Slip Off. I Prefer to Do This with No Shoes or Socks on; However, You May Choose to Wear Your Shoes To Start with (definitely in public restrooms) Until You Build up confidence.

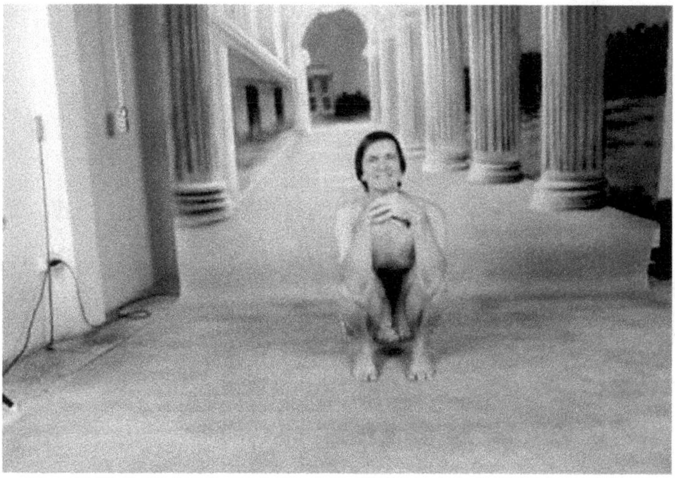

Advanced method of squatting on a western toilet:

This is not needed, however, it helps to build core strength. Stand on the bowl rim put your arms out straight. Next, slowly lower down to a squatting position. The slower, the better the workout. When you are finished with your business, put your palms on the bowl rim in front of you, obviously not a public toilet, lift up your torso with your arm and core strength, with control swing or slide your feet toward the front of you and on the floor. Pending on your physical abilities this may take a while to perfect. My core muscle group was not strong in that way it took me more than 6 months.

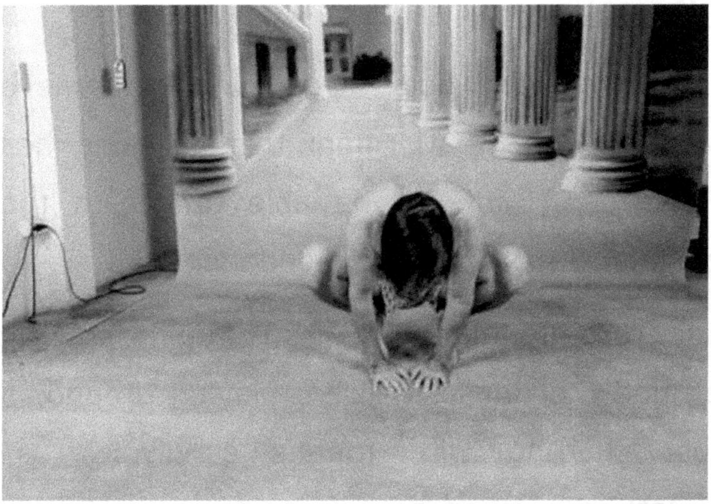

Alternatives:

Okay, I know what you're thinking, some of you say wow great! I think this is a good idea. However, I will not be able to get in that position. I have 2 recommendations.

1st recommendation, when you're working around the house, garden, playing around, or just chatting with friends simply do the squatting position as long as you can. Even if it's only for 1 minute that will be a start. When I 1st started it was only 30 seconds for me when I spoke with friends in Peru South America. My calves were very tight, however, with a little time and practice the rewards came quickly.

2nd recommendation you could get a toilet squatting platform. This will make it not so extreme to go for a Western-style seating position to full on squatting position. Check out the video link at the http://backpainreliefin45minutes.com/, it will explain many more benefits than the few that I had touched on. I highly recommend you watch the video even if you do not need the aid of the platform. It goes over in much more visual details of the benefits of the squatting to your health than I can cover in the scope of this book.

Inducing the Relaxation Response

Inducing the relaxation response is a phrase coined by Dr. Herbert Benson, he is a researcher that discovered that a short as eight weeks of meditation 15 minutes per day can literally change your DNA structure!

Basically, this refers to meditation, in no way as this meant to offend or put off anybody. If you have a different spiritual belief or religious following than only do your practice that goes along with your lifestyle. The following is what really works for me after many years of trying different things.

Here's a short list of just some of the many benefits.

- ✓ Increased health
- ✓ increased happiness
- ✓ more control
- ✓ think more clearly
- ✓ create less stress
- ✓ more energized
- ✓ eat better
- ✓ more calm state
- ✓ weight loss

WOW! meditation what a great thing, there are hundreds of books on meditating. I have studied many. I have even gone as far as taking 10 day, vegetarian, no talking, 6 hours per day meditation retreats. I'm not suggesting you need to do that; however what I will give you here, is a very simple easy to do meditation program, you can learn in a few minutes.

A few minutes of meditation every day can change your life, really it has mine. I believe it is the number one self-improvement thing that you can do for yourself, **PERIOD!** Actually meditation is very simple.

Find a nice quiet private place for yourself. Don't worry about being in full lotus Yogi position, just sit comfortably for you. I sit on a soft rug on my heels, my hands in my lap, my back and shoulders arched back a little bit. You don't want to be slouched over or leaning. A good posture is one when you look dignified, sitting like a king or queen; you are relaxed, however, very self-confident.

1. You will want an anchor just like a boat on the shore something to keep you tethered and

focused I have found a very simple way to do that. Close your eyes, focus on your breathing, follow the breathing going in your nostrils and into your lungs seeing the number 1 tumbling as it goes into your nostril. Then follow the number 1 as it exhaling leaving your lungs and nostrils.

2. The next inhale and exhale as 2. Etc. etc. etc.

Okay, simple enough, right? Yeah, it's true it simple enough, however, what you may find is your mind wanders, and you lose track of the numbers, that is very normal. I would be very surprised if you could just count to 10 without losing track. Just refocus on counting and the breath. Here is a little trick I found very helpful, on Day 1, Just meditate for 60 seconds. That's it! Just 60 seconds. 1 minutes only. Everybody can do that. Then on day 2, 2 minutes only. Then on day 3, 3 minutes only and so on and so on. Okay, now work your way up to 15 minutes per day. It depends on how quick you breathed ideally counting to 50 should be about 15 minutes, however, for some that can be as much as 75 breaths. Maximum meditation results our when you breathe deep and slow without any sound on the inhale and next. You could go for the expert level, put a little pause at the end of your exhale and inhale. When you meditate 15 minutes per day for 30 days, you will see vast changes in your life. What I found was a vast change in my state. I was calmer, more relaxed; I focus much better. Personally I do 15 minutes the very first thing in the morning, and then I do 15 minutes the very last thing just before I go to sleep. This is a great way to create an amazing day! :-)

At one time in my life, I was meditating 3hrs a day! Wow! is right. OK, a little secret, 15 minutes a day of quality mediation is all you need. Life is meant to be creative, active and social! enjoy yourself and others!

It seemed to me things happen in my life much

easier, stuff that I want or things I wanted to happen just happened with little or no effort on my part.

Enjoy!

Get out of the box! Move your body

In our Western world today, our movements have been limited and restricted. We sit in chairs, we sit in the car; we sit on the couch. Many First World people are limited, or we don't have a type of sports for physical movement practices. Most of the people around the world have a range of motion for their bodies much larger than the First World. For example, they sit on the floor; they climb trees to pick food, walk to the market, tend the garden. I have lived in countries like Peru, Mexico, and Thailand, and I have met people there over 90 years old that get up and down as they still sit on the floor, and take care of all their own needs to cook cleaning and doing their own laundry by hand. My recommendation to you is to turn off the TV, roll around on the floor, go play with the kids or grandkids get on the grass, take off your shoes, take up a sport, start doing your favorite exercises....

As you can see, most everyone can do these simple movements in this back pain relief book. Don't worry about being perfect, just do the best that you can do at that moment. Don't push yourself and don't hurt yourself. You may feel a little pain but not a lot, take it slow and easy. You will get better each and every day. As you can see or maybe already experienced the simple steps enclosed here have quick benefits. There may be a few areas in your life that you could change to serve your back and life health better. Once you're feeling good again. It is important to keep up with some kind of physical maintenance program, yoga, Pilates and also add some sports or physical activities in your life. If you find it hard to get started or stay on a good physical routine, I would recommend you check out a rebounder or mini trampoline.

Rebounder:

I find that 20 minutes replace my 1 hour bike ride, yoga or swimming sessions with a full body work out. I find it very easy to do, here are some of the many benefits.

- Improves spinal alignment and posture, regular rebounding, has been shown to help relieve joint, back and neck pain over time.
- Deeper and more relaxed sleep
- Mental synapses are improved and increased

- Improves the body's response to PMS for women
- Helps to reduce the number of flues, colds and stomach ailments
- Has been shown to reduce cellular atrophy due to aging.
- Reaction time necessary for proprioceptors located in joints is improved, transmission of nerve impulses along the myelin sheaths to and from the brain, spinal cord and muscle fibers is improved
- Allow the brain to respond better to the vestibular apparatus inside the inner ear which helps improve balance in the body over time.
- The digestive peristalsis is re-calibrated and improved by a regular rebound practice.
- The up and down action of rebounding causes large muscle groups to contract which makes a rhythmic compression of

every artery and vein in the body. Helps to increase circulation, increase blood flow and oxygenation of tissues which in turn helps to reduce blood pressure and puts less strain on your heart muscle.

- Improves lung capacity and respiration
- The height of the arterial pressure that's needed for exercise is reduced
- Decreases the amount of time blood pressure rises after intense exercise
- Helps to lower blood clots that could stagnate and pool in the veins , which cause edema in the extremities.
- Bouncing longer than twenty minutes at medium intensity 3 or more times per week increases the mitochondria within the cells and that helps endurance athletes in particular.
- Allows the body to achieve an alkaline pH in the body easier.

- Helps to reduce the number of free form cholesterol in the body as well as levels of triglycerides.

- Lower low-density lipoprotein (bad) in the blood and increases high-density lipoprotein (good) holding off the incidence of coronary artery disease.

- Cellular repair and tissue repair are enhanced

- The G-force that occurs on the body due to acceleration helps strengthen the musculoskeletal system.

- About 85% of the impact on the joints are mitigated unlike doing jump rope or running. I personally do not like to run it hurts my knees.

- The ability to manage your BMI (body mass index) improves as well as your muscle to fat ratio.

- Increased circulation and oxygenation for improved organ and tissue health
- Because bouncing helps to increase cellular circulation that allows the capillary count in the muscles to increase which then diminishes the distance between these capillaries and other target cells in the body.
- Causes the heart to become stronger over time. Which pumps more blood.
- Regular bouncing over time helps to reduce the resting heart rate of most individuals.
- The acceleration and deceleration helps to strengthen the heart even after heart surgery.
- Helps to create the a healthier red blood cell that's able to function at higher efficiency
- Over time rebounding helps to reset your resting metabolism and metabolic rate so

you burn more calories even when you're not exercising

- Young and old can do it
- Detoxifies
- Strengthens every cell in the body
- Increases bone density,

Most importantly it is **FUN!**

Video Series

Don't forget it is important to enjoy yourself! Be aware of your body and mind, and they will take care of you and give you great rewards.

Here is the direct link to BackPainRelief.com it contains the how to videos and other helpful information. NOTE: to access the video you will want to put in the password "happy".

Hydrotherapy

Everyone knows that you get relief from the super hot as you can bath. About 3 cups of Epson salt and a small box of baking soda and a little lavender oil from Sequim Washington really it does the trick for me. Also if you can gain access to a hot bubbly Jacuzzi you can focus the Jets on the sore spots, it can be most wonderful. These two ideas can relaxes your muscles and can give some pain relief.

Now the Real Magic Water Therapy:

How Would You like to Get the Following Benefits?

*Stimulate your immune system

*release stiffness and relaxed muscles for greater healing

*deeper sleep

*better body fluid circulation

*pump out toxins

*pump in oxygen

*refresh yourself

*clarify your mind

*breathe deeper, similar to good exercise

*feel fantastic energized and more alive!

Do you remember jumping into a cold Lake, River, or Ocean on a hot day, remember how you felt? WOW! What a feeling!

Here's the trick: Shower Therapy

It is very simple to do, but most definitely will be a little challenging for you at first. But, I'm telling you the rewards are well worth it. Go experiences for yourself.

1. 30 to 60 Seconds of the Hottest Water You Can Take.

2. 30 to 60 Seconds of the Coldest Water You Can Take.

3. Work your way up to five sets :-)

4. Always finish with a cold, attempt to get all of your body.

Ideally you want to work your way up to 60 seconds, and then five rounds. And when you and make sure it's a nice long cold. I usually do a couple minutes of cold in the end. At first do what you can. If you've never done anything like this, it will be a "BIG SHOCK" pun intended :-). When I first started doing this, I screamed like a teenage girl for the first couple days. Gradually day by day increase the length of time until you get up to 60 second mark. Also note you can target their areas that are giving you the most pain, alternating back and forth with the hot and cold. That will increase the circulation in those areas, giving you some relief.

A six weeks hospital trials showed increases in plasma concentration, T cell helpers and lymphocytes. That is an amazing thing to do and shows how you have control over making your body heal itself.

I found this concept many years ago and to this day I still use some form of it. My friends think I'm crazy; though, I mostly take a cold shower now. My friends who have switched feel the benefits also :-).

Some Swedish families still follow the old tradition today by putting their babies outside for naps in the cold air! What they found is those children are more resistant to disease and sleep deeper.

Massages

With the above First 4 positions, I return me back to working health in a matter of one week. However, later I found that Thai massage can greatly improve the body's ability to heal quicker by opening up the blood flow of any blocked energy passages and besides it feels great! You will have to invest some money in Thai massages as they are not cheap. This, however, is well worth the money if you have it. The alternative is to see if there is a local group of Thais living in your city. Contact them to see if they know any masseuses. If not, buy a book on Thai massage and have a friend do some work on you :-).

Seeing Is Believing

How you see yourself, what you constantly think about is a reflection of your well-being.

DEHYPNOTIZE YOURSELF!

Negative thoughts have exactly the same effect upon our behavior as the negative thoughts implanted into the mind of a hypnotized subject by a professional hypnotist.

Normally for things to come into our life we see them in our minds first. Unfortunately, many of us repeat disempowering word phrases patterns or visions. Example seeing yourself not being able to work because of your back pain, seeing yourself not being able to perform a certain job function because of your back pain.

What we I understand

PSYCHO CYBERNETICS

I once asked a friend of mine how he became a multimillionaire and very successful, healthy businessman. He told me in his mid-30s he was working in a warehouse and knew that there was more to life than this. Then he read this book called Psycho Cybernetics by Maxwell Maltz. That changed his whole life :-). Recommend recommended reading if you find the subject interesting. So what does it say?

Basically set aside 30 minutes per day visualizing the perfect you, the super healthy you, the more successful you, the happier you, the one in crazy love you, the one with lots of money you. And any other thing that would you like to see changed or make improvements on.

I know this may sound a little odd to do this; that's what I thought at first. Then I read where the Olympic athletes and other top athletes stopped working out so much and put time into visualization, seeing themself perform perfectly in the events that they wanted. They got better results! And as I said my friend who's lives an incredible lifestyle. Then when I started to do it in my own life, AMAZING results. It is fun, simple, and that results will astound you. I live my dream life.

The following quotes are by Maxwell Maltz.

"Your nervous system cannot tell the difference between an imagined experience and a 'real' experience."

Why not imagine you successful?

"Imagine how you would feel if you were already the sort of personality you want to be. and feeling good because of it. see yourself acting calmly and deliberately, acting with confidence and courage—and feeling expansive and confident because you are."

"This exercise builds new 'memories' or stored data into your mid-brain and central nervous system. It builds a new image of self. After practicing it for a time, you will be surprised to find yourself 'acting differently,' more or less automatically and spontaneously— 'without trying."-- Maxwell Maltz

For take out a piece of paper and a pen, and write down the perfect you. So get to it go visualize the perfect you in all aspects, not just your physical body!

Healing Back Pain:

the Mind-Body Connection

Tension Mitosis Syndrome TMS

Tension Mitosis Syndrome Is Groundbreaking Research Put out by Dr. Sarno. Dr. Sarno talks about how to identify stress and other psychological factors associated with back pain. Points out how many of his clients have gone through healing themselves without exercise or physical therapy? Cannot be true? It is a must-read, even if you get a little benefit from this book and Dr. Sarno's concepts. It can greatly benefit you.

*Why self-motivated and successful people are prone to TMS

*How anxiety and repressed anger trigger muscle spasms

*How people "train themselves' to experience back pain

*How you may get relief from back pain within two to six weeks by recognizing TMS and its causes

I don't agree with everything in the book; however, I find a lot of valid points and suggestions in the book. I think it's a very good read in your arsenal to reverse and eliminate your back pain issues. Read it for yourself and take the parts that work for you. I believe it's well worth your time to check out.

Super foods

I have taken as much as $600 a month of nutritional supplements. Crazy Ha, heck that is the payment on a nice vacation house in Florida!

Anyway with all the years of trying many different things I came up with two products that I would highly recommend you get on as soon as possible. You don't need all the massive amounts of nutritional stuff. Just eat well and try out the following two items.

Number one:

Dr. Schulze's Superfood plus. It is organic whole food, herbal, vitamin and mineral product. I learned of this product when I saw a man of 118 years old who has been taking it for more than 30 years. And he claims it's one of his reasons for living so long outside the fact he walks one-mile every day. The reason I picked Dr. Scholl's is because very old established business, lots of success stories, and it's a great value for what you get.

Number two:

BodyBoost colostrum. The Superfood Extraordinaire. Before I found colostrum I used to take human growth hormone supplement, outside the fact it was very expensive and they were some side effects there were some great benefits to it. But they have been all replaced an even more with amazing whole colostrum which is just a Superfood. Colostrum is the only supplement you can take to add back antibodies and immune factors. It has more than 100 beneficial components, growth factors, cytokine precursors that you can't get from any other supplement. Very potent antiaging and broad spectrum probiotics in a whole food form. On the website, they talk about clinical studies of enhance stamina, increase in lean body mass, anaerobic power, performance time and increase sexual function. The reason I choose BodyBoost colostrum is they are one of the leaders in bringing modern colostrum to the public. They have been around a long time, and they appear to have very good quality, never had an issue. And the big thing is there colostrum comes from the very first milking after the birth of the calf. You get the premium stuff.

Some things I noticed for myself, I think much clearer, have a lot more energy, and rarely get sick. Colds and flu never really visit our home, even though the neighborhood may have it. Anyways go try it out, and you'll see what I'm talking about. You will thank me, please feel free to send me an email that would be wonderful! :-).

You can go to their websites for more details, and both are available on Amazon. Both of these will make a huge difference in their health. I don't need to go over all the benefits here in this book you can research for yourself all the many benefits on the information directly from the manufacture. One thing I will say is I like to buy things in bulk powder that's my personal preference. I have more control of the product, and it always seems to be a lot cheaper that way. However, sometimes capsules are very convenient, and we seem to have some on hand most of the time.

"***It is health that is real wealth and not pieces of gold and silver.***"

-Mahatma Gandhi

Wrapping It Up,

Okay, that's it see how simple it is just a quick review.

- Take up to two days rest in bed if necessary, don't forget the popcorn! :-)
- Drink two glasses of water upon waking, then at least 6 more daily
- Start meditating, 60 seconds on the first day :-)
- Drink a smoothie or vegetable juice with

your Superfood supplement

- Visualizing what you really want
- start the four main positions
- Learn and implement the breathing technique
- hot and cold water therapy twice a day
- Do the exercises for at least four days after you feel pretty good
- Make some life changing choices if you so desire
- Do a weekly back care tune-up
- Start a daily exercise routine
- Spend quality time with loved ones

Biography

Marcus D. Norman, I was born in Michigan 1960. I have a mother that tweaked her back at work more than 35 years ago. After five surgeries and different therapy's, the doctor told me that my mother would've been better off not having any of the surgeries. She would have most likely had a full recovery! Because of all the medical intervention mother never fully recovered and is on pain medication which affects her life in many ways. She finds it difficult to focus and do simple tasks, swimming which she loved is now a walk around the pool.

From that point forward, I became much interested in our bodies, and how to best take care of them.

Up until that point I was a verified couch potato! Junk food and Movies!!!

I love to study and learn. So, I discovered yoga over 30 years ago. Have studied many modality of the body mechanics and how to optimize function. Have taught and did demonstrations. Study with some of the world's best instructors. Anthony Carlisi, John Friend, David Swenson, Tias Little and Pete Egoscue to name a few. Active in outdoor playing; like scuba, sailing, snow skiing, hiking mountains. Example Machu Picchu in Cusco Peru (14,050 ft above sea level) have done that 3 day hike five different times. For me, it is like winning a Gold Medal, what an amazing experience to reach this ancient city. Three 5,000 mile motorcycle trip thru Mexico, Flying

Hang glider, Ultra lights, Para-gliders, sailplanes, Cycling.

Have lived and traveled to 18 countries. I appreciate other cultures and customs. Love to be outdoors. My diet is mostly veggie juice's, rice, fruits, vegetables seafood and eat little meat. Crazy for Thai food!!!

basic Life philosophy..."**LIFE IS GOOD!**"

Thank you so much for purchasing my little book. I really appreciate your positive reviews; they can be left at Amazon. I would like to make this even better, to help you and others further on their health journey.

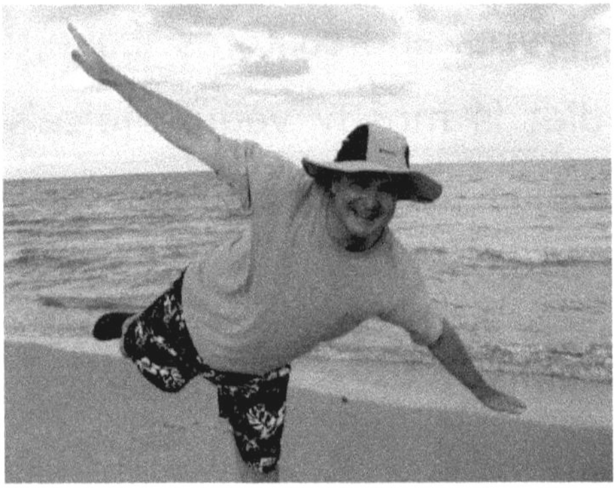

Please send any comments or questions to MarcusDNorman@gmail.com

Oh! another Thing,

share your thoughts on Facebook and Twitter. If you believe the book is worth sharing, would you take a few seconds to let your friends know about it? You could mention the FREE how to videos series. If it turns out to make a difference in their lives, they'll be forever grateful to you. As I will.

All the best, Marcus D. Norman

Recommended Reads

The MELT Method: A Breakthrough Self-Treatment System to Eliminate Chronic Pain, Erase the Signs of Aging, and Feel Fantastic in Just 10 Minutes a Day!

Healing Back Pain: The Mind-Body Connection

Foundation: Redefine Your Core, Conquer Back Pain, and Move with Confidence

The Mindbody Prescription: Healing the Body, Healing the Pain

8 Steps to a Pain-Free Back: Natural Posture Solutions for Pain in the Back, Neck, Shoulder, Hip, Knee, and Foot

Pain Free: A Revolutionary Method for Stopping Chronic Pain

The Trigger Point Therapy Workbook: Your Self-Treatment Guide for Pain Relief

I would like to give a very special thanks to Sandy, for the endless list of Wonderful Life Adventures and improvements she continues to give to all, she is a true friend. Love you.

And to my incredible wife. For her patients, support, and great cooking. Also, my inspirational daughter.

"Life is truly Good"

Disclaimer: the information contained in this book is based on the experience and research of the author The author of this book dos not dispense medical advice or prescribe the use of any technique as a form of treatment for physical, emotional, or medical problems. You should seek the advice of a physician. The intent of the authors is only to offer information of a general nature to help you in your quest for wellbeing. In the event, you use any of the information in this book for yourself, which is your constitutional right, the author and the publisher assume no responsibility for your actions.

Some of the persons names mentioned in this book have been changed to protect the privacy of the individuals. The names in the testimonial sections have not been changed and are authentic.

Notes

The End

www.ingramcontent.com/pod-product-compliance
Lightning Source LLC
Chambersburg PA
CBHW050539280326
41933CB00011B/1640
9780615973647